SUBSTANCE MISUSE

AWARENESS HANDBOOK

FD Wuriee

author shall in no event be held liable to any party for any direct, indirect, punitive, special, incidental or other consequential damages arising directly or indirectly from any use of this material, which is provided "as is", and without warranties. As always, the advice of a competent professional in the subject and or field of the subject should be sought. The author do not warrant the performance, or effectiveness of this book.

Page

Chapter 1

1.0 Introduction to Substance Misuse

Substance Misuse is a common term which differs to substance addiction. In this chapter you will learn about the basic sectors of substance misuse. Topics to be covered as follow:

(a) What is substance misuse?

(b) Commonly misused substances

(c) Substance use and misuse.

(d) Abuse and addiction

(e) Substance use disorder.

(f) Signs of substance misuse

(g) Behavioural symptoms

(h) Physical Symptoms

(i) Psychological Symptoms

(j) Reasons Behind substance misuse

What is Substance misuse?

Misuse of a substance is the use of alcohol, illicit drugs or prescription or over the counter drugs in such a manner that they are not intended to be consumed and may be dangerous to you and those around you. People may use drugs once, rarely or daily and they may continue to experience drug use disorder. A disorder of substance use happens when alcohol or medication impair your fitness and act in your daily life. Substances can be something you insert into your body and can affect the way your brain function. These changes can affect your perception, mood, thinking and behaviour.

Commonly misuse substances.

These include alcohol, beer, wine, distilled spirit. Nicotine products such as cigarette, cigars, e-cigarette, and smokeless tobacco.

Marijuana including synthetic Marijuana, K2, Spice.

Drugs such as heroin, codeine, oxycodone (oxycontin), morphine, hydrocodone (Vicodin), fentanyl, and hydromorphone hydrochloride.

Benzodiazepines, including diazepam (Valium), lorazepam (Ativan), alprazolam (Xanax) and clonazepam (klonopin)

Over the counter such as cold or cough medicines. Other substances, including cocaine, amphetamines, methamphetamine, and other stimulants. Misuse is not inherently limited to one substance. Polysubstance usage refers to the consuming at the same time more than one drug. This could be deliberate such as combining a drug with alcohol to intensify the effect.

Substance Use and Misuse

Experts agree that the line between drug use and addiction blurs as prolong use affect particular life facets. For example, if daily use result in one of the following, the person is likely to have a drug abuse problem

- Health complications as a result of substance abuse
- Inability to carry out daily responsibilities.
- Physical dependence
- Withdrawal symptoms if usage stops.
- Craving for drug or alcohol

Drug misuse can also lead to substance abuse, although this is not necessarily the case. Drug addiction and drug abuse are not the same.

Abuse and Addiction

Addiction doesn't begin overnight. It takes time to gain tolerance for the drug of choice. Develop cravings for drugs and suffer complications related to the use of controlled narcotics. Drug misuse always begins first. The symptoms is the failure to resist alcohol. Someone who deals with substance abuse may have many issues that affect those with addiction but may be able to avoid consuming all drugs without problems for a long time. However, an addict cannot stay away from his or her choice of drugs and other substances despite a strong urge to stop using them.

Substance Use Disorder

A disorder of substance use happens when the use of alcohol or another substance (drug) causes health complications or problems at work, school, or home. This disorder is also called substance abuse. The precise cause of substance use disorder is unspecified. Some causes may be Genes, drug action, social control, personal pain, Fear, Depression, environmental stress.

Many people who develop drug use problems have addiction, attention deficit disorder, Post traumatic stress disorder (PTSD), or other psychiatric problems. Stressful or unstable lifestyles and poor self- esteem are also widespread. Children who grow up watching their parents take drugs may have a high chance of having substance use problems later in life for both environmental and genetic factors.

Identifying the symptoms of addiction is the first step in helping yourself or leading those you care for to rehabilitate. It is also crucial to provide an awareness of the symptoms of addiction. There are behavioural, physical, and psychological symptoms of addictions.

Behavioural Symptoms: Symptoms include a person's external relationship with the environment, while medical signs refer to the appearance of side effects by the body due to the existence of substances in the system. Behavioural signs include but not limited to: -

- **Obsessive thoughts and action** – in this case, acquiring and consuming drugs are the key goals in life, while any other responsibilities including job, family or education are ignored.
- **Disregard of Harm Caused** – Since substance misuse causes physical and mental trauma to individuals and their loved ones, a person dealing with addiction tends to use narcotics or alcohol.
- **Loss Of Control** – Even in the face of wanting to stop or reduce their drug use, the person cannot do so.

- **Staying in Denial** – When approached, the person struggling with addiction will reject or reduce their use of drugs. To escape having to justify themselves to others, a person will do drugs in secret.

Drug misuse cannot stay secret for a long time. Its effect is too drastic, and people who use drugs will quickly spin out of control.

Physical Symptoms: Physical symptoms of addictions can manifest as side effects of use, overdose, or because of withdrawal. It can be very difficult for anyone to identify the clinical symptoms source, but serious consequences may require emergency medical attention.

> **Physical signs of addictions** are as follow: Enlarge or small pupil, Sudden weight gain or loss, Bloodshot eyes, insomnia, unusual body odours, Poor physical coordination, Looking unkempt, slurred speech.

> **Signs of overdose** are as follow: Drowsiness or trouble walking, Agitation, Aggression or violent behaviour, Difficulty breathing, Nausea and vomiting, Hallucinations, Delusions, Loss of consciousness.

Withdrawal Symptoms are as follow: Shakiness, trembling and jumpiness, loss of appetite, Nausea and vomiting, Depression, Insomnia and fatigue, Headaches and fever, Confusion and hallucinations, Seizures.

Psychological Symptoms: Drug misuse also affects the psychological status of the victim. If they are in the grasp of addiction, the individual does not know or notice these dangers.

Psychological signs are as follow: Anxiousness, inattentiveness, lack of motivation, irritability or angry outbursts, Changes in personality or attitude, Emotional and mental withdrawing from people, Sudden mood swings, unexpected paranoia.

Reasons behind Substance Misuse

Different types of substances abuse can arise for many different causes. Although each addiction is different, and the severity may vary from drug to substance, there are several general causes people can become addicted to the substance. The causes are as follow: -

Depression- Many people who are struggling with depression do not get adequate medication for this issue. Many coping with depression appear to self-medicate the effect of depression with alcohol, marijuana, cocaine, and various other mind altering drugs

Fitting In – Peer pressure encourages people to do things they wouldn't have done, either to appease their peers or to want to be appreciate.

Self-Medicating – Stress, fear, recurring discomfort, undiagnosed psychiatric disorders, extreme depression, isolation, trauma are some responsible for addiction. These are all reasons that people will self-medicated by mind altering drugs to deal with what they feel or don't want to feel

Curiosity – Often, people feel curiosity towards substances which later leads to substance misuse.

Prescribed Medication – Some people believe that when a doctor issues them a prescription, the drug they are taking is healthy to take without any effects. Unfortunately, addictive substance medications are highly toxic and can serve as a pathway to other drugs such as heroin.

Chapter 2

2.0 Overview of Substance

Introduction: Substances can include substances, alcohol and other stuff that is injurious to health. This chapter will give you an idea of what substances are and how they work. A clear idea of this will help you in the case of substance misuse management and prevention. Topics to be covered in this chapter as follow: -

Types of Substances

- Stimulus
- Depressants
- Hallucinogens
- Opium related painkillers

Legal and Illegal Substances. Illegal substances Overview

Effects of Different Substances

- Alcohol
- Crystal Meth
- Anabolic Steroids
- Benzodiazepines
- Buprenorphine

- Cannabis (Marijuana)

- Cocaine

- Ecstasy (MDMA)

- Heroin

- LSD

- Nicotine

- Solvents

Health Risks of Substances

Types Of Substances: All substances have some kind of effect on your mental health. They affect the way you see things, your mood, and your behaviour. If you take a substance, it is difficult to predict how you will react to a substance. You may react differently to the same substance at different times or in different situations. There are four main classes of substances, grouped according to their major effects, and a few compounds that do not fall neatly into either grouping. These four classes are –

- Stimulants (for example Cocaine)

- Depressants (for example alcohol)

- Opium related pain killer (for example heroin)

- Hallucinogens (for example LSD)

Stimulants – Stimulants speed up the messages between the brain and the body. This can cause:

- Heart to beat faster.
- Agitation
- Blood pressure to go up.
- Reduce appetite.
- Sleeplessness
- Body temperature to go up – leading to heat exhaustion or even stroke.

Stimulants make you feel more awake, more alert, more optimistic or more energetic. Larger doses can induce fear, panic, epilepsy, stomach cramps and paranoia. Some examples of stimulants are.

- Amphetamines (speed and ice)
- Caffeine
- Cocaine
- Ecstasy(MDMA–Methylenedioxy Methamphetamine)
- Nicotine (tobacco)

Depressants – Depressants slow down signals from your brain and your body. They don't actually make you feel sad.

They slower messages affect your concentration and your ability to respond to what's happening around you. Tiny doses of depressants can make you feel relaxed, calm and less inhibited. Larger doses can lead to sleepiness, vomiting and nausea, Unconsciousness and even death. Examples of depressants include.

- Alcohol
- Cannabis
- Ketamine
- Ghb (Gamma-hydroxybutyrate)
- Opioids (heroin, morphine, codeine)
- Benzodiazepines (minor tranquilisers such as Valium)

Hallucinogens – Hallucinogens alter the sense of reality - you may hallucinate. Your senses are skewed, and the way you see, hear, taste, smell or feel is different. For instance, you can see or hear objects that aren't there, or you may have strange thoughts or feelings. Larger doses can induce hallucinations, loss of memory, depression, anxiety, elevated heart rate, paranoia, fear, and aggression. Examples of Hallucinogens are.

- Cannabis

- Ketamine

- PCP (phencyclidine)

- LSD (Lysergic acid diethylamide)

- Psilocybin (magic mushrooms)

Opium Related Pain Killers – Opioids, also known as opiate, are a class of substances found in the opium poppy plant. Opioids function in a multitude of ways, manipulating various molecules in the brain to provide a high sensation. When someone uses prescription medications, they are usually referred to as pain relievers and they are referred to as pain killers. They make you feel.

- A rush of pleasure

- Drowsy

- In a dreamy state

They are very dangerous at high doses. They are addictive substances.

2.1 Legal and Illegal Substances

Legal medications should be purchased over the counter or prescription by a licenced doctor. Illegal medications cannot be lawfully made, purchase or marketed. Certain other substances are legal in some cases, but they are prohibited when they abused. These variations between medications can be misleading.

Many substances such as marijuana, caffeine, and nicotine are safe but may be subject to age, place of use, driving and point of scale limitations.

2.2 Illegal Substances Overview

Medicine is a substance that affects the way the body works. If a substance is listed as criminal, this means that it is banned by law. Different illicit substances have different effects on individuals, and several factors affect these effects. That makes them unpredictable and dangerous, particularly for young people. The effects of a substance are influenced by:

- The type of substance which is used.
- Number of substances which is consumed.
- Where the person is and when the substance is being used
- What the person is doing while using the substances
- Individual characteristics such as body size and health vulnerabilities

- How many different substances are taken at one time.

Effects Of Different Substances – The possible mental health effects of the most used substance is listed below.

Alcohol. Alcohol is legal but it is the most toxic of commonly used substances. Moderate use is not usually a problem. The long-term effects are associated with drinking a lot over a long period of time. These effects will go away if you stop drinking. The short-term effect of alcohol are-

- Feeling relaxed and more sociable
- Feeling subdued, so that you drink more to recreate the pleasure effects.
- Large amounts – uninhibited behaviour or aggression

Long term effects of alcohol are-

- Memory loss
- Addiction
- Poor concentration
- Difficulty thinking clearly.
- Difficulty problem solving

Crystal Meth – Amphetamines are a category of substances that differ in how effective they are and how lawfully classified they are. The symptoms of crystal meth are comparable to cracking cocaine, but they last longer. If you have a mental health disorder, you are more likely to have harmful effects. Short term effects are: Reduced tiredness, increase energy and confidence, Increase attention and alertness.

Long term effect of crystal meth is- Agitation, Aggression, Confusion, Psychosis and Paranoia

Anabolic Steroids – these are used to improve muscle mass and boost athletic ability. They're sluggish to respond and they don't trigger instant buzz like most stimulants. They are class C medications, lawfully available only by prescription by a pharmacist. Many sports organisations are prohibited from using them.

Short- and long-term effects are: Excitement, Aggression, Confusion, Depression, Sleeping problems, Increase energy, Competitiveness and Dramatic mood swings

Benzodiazepines – these are prescribed for anxiety and sleeping pills. It is illegal to take them without a prescription written for you.

Negative effects are Agitation, Aggression and Hostility

Positive effects are: Reduce tension and anxiety, Clear thinking, Feeling calm and relaxed.

Buprenorphine – Buprenorphine and methadone are both prescription substances that are used to treat heroin addiction.

Short- and long-term effects are: Depression, Loss of libido, Feelings of detachment Hallucinations and other psychotic symptoms

Cannabis (Marijuana) – people take cannabis as a way of relaxing and getting high. The results that you feel will largely depend on

- Whether you are used to taking the substance
- How much you take.
- Your genes
- The type of cannabis you use.

If you develop anxiety and depression, you are more likely to experience negative side effects. Short term effects are Hunger, Talkative, Feeling relaxed, Finding things very funny and laughing a lot and Feeling excited by the things you see, hear and feel

High doses may cause: Forgetfulness, Distress and confusion, Psychotic experiences, and Distorted perceptions.

Long term effects are Depression in later life, if you use it a lot as a teenager and Long lasting symptoms of psychosis that may be diagnosed as schizophrenia

Cocaine – Cocaine comes in two forms. Cocaine powder which is snorted and crack cocaine which is smoked. Both forms may be injected. Cocaine is notoriously impure and often contains other substances.

Short term effects: Full of energy, feeling confident and feeling wide awake

High doses may cause: Hallucinations, Depression and Suicidal thoughts.

Long term effects are: anxiety, depression, paranoia, panic attacks, irreversible brain damage, worsening of pre-existing mental health problems

Ecstasy (MDMA) – Ecstasy pills are notoriously impure and frequently contain substances other than MDMA. While ecstasy is a stimulant, it has different effects than other stimulants because it induces feelings of empathy rather than euphoria.

Short term effects are: Feeling happy and feeling of empathy, openness and caring.

Long term effects are Anxiety, Confusion, Loss of Confidence, Agitation and teeth clenching, panic attacks after repeated use, depression which does not respond to antidepressants, Hallucinations and paranoia after repeated high doses.

Heroin – Heroin is an antidepressant that is usually prescribed as diamorphine. The primary symptoms include the relaxation of suffering and euphoria, but also exhaustion. It's addictive and it's leading many people to violence for finance their use of it.

Short term effects are Insomnia, lethargy, drowsiness, talkativeness, loss of appetite, and a rush of pleasure followed by calm, warm, dreamy contentment

Long term effects are Loss of appetite, apathy, neglect of personal safety and hygiene, generalised pain when the level of substance in your system drops

LSD – LSD is a synthetic compound that was first produced in the 1940s. It produces random and often terrifying results, such as poor trips, which can be postponed. The effects of magic mushrooms are like LSD.

Short term effects are Hallucinations, Altered sense of space and time, feeling that you can fly, Anxiety (associated with bad trip), detachment from surroundings, feeling panicky (associated with bad trip)

Long term effects are Flashbacks of bad trips, when you feel you are relieving them, likely to worsen existing symptoms of schizophrenia.

Nicotine – Normally you will not suffer the mental health consequences of nicotine use. However, it is highly addictive and stopping nicotine can have negative effects. While you are taking part in nicotine reduction program, substances such as bupropion (zybang), varenicline (champix), or benzodiazepine can be given to help you deal with withdrawal symptoms.

Solvents – Solvents, glues, and aerosols can affect the pulse and cause death. Repeating sniffing can induce a hangover effect, making you pale, very sleepy, forgetful, and unable to focus. They are primarily used by young people, normally only for a limited time. It is illegal to market glues to young people under the age of 18 if you believe they will be using them to sniff.

Short term effects are Dizziness, aggression, depression, mood swings, euphoria, loss of inhibition, feelings similar to getting drunk, pseudo hallucinations -hallucinations that you know are not real) and feeling unreal

2.3 Health Risks of Substances

In 2017, 3,284 substance related deaths (DRDS) occurred in the UK using the European Monitoring Centre for Narcotics and Drugs Abuse (EMCDDA) definition, which is death caused directly by the ingestion of at least one illegal substance.

The substance related death rate per million population in the UK using the EMCDDA concept was the highest reported at 76 per million. The death rate in Scotland was 229 per million in 2017, the highest recorded in Europe that year. The prevalence of hepatitis C among people who inject substances surveyed in England, Wales, and Northern Ireland in 2018 was 55%. This is the biggest number of the last decade. In Scotland, the prevalence reported from 2017 to 2018 was 57%

Chapter 3

3.0 Prevention and Awareness

Introduction: Substance misuse can have far reaching implications. In this chapter you will learn about the prevention principles and methods that could be relevant solutions. Topics to be covered are as follow:

Why is Prevention Important?

Principles of Prevention

- Intervention
- Managing Prevention Programs

Ideas for Substance Awareness Projects

- Discussions
- Fairs and Displays
- Pamphlets
- Videos
- Performances
- Media Campaign
- Conferences
- Other Projects

Financial Resources

3.0 Why Is Prevention Important?

Substance abuse is a leading source of sickness and mortality in the world. In addition, substance abuse can have severe repercussions and worsen existing individual and social inequities.

Substance abuse can lead to a decline in physical and mental health and social issues on an individual level. Therefore, a comprehensive approach to manage substance use and support the population's health, well-being and productivity must include prevention. It is especially crucial in rural areas, where many young people and adolescents are marginalised and poor. Evidence based preventative methods that are implemented over time and address various age groups and communities can have a significant impact on rural youths and adolescents' health and well-being.

The primary goal of substance use prevention is to help nonsubstance users avoid or delay substance use initiation. For those who are already substance users, prevention seeks to minimise the likelihood of developing substance use disorders (example, dependence). The prevention also has a broader purpose:

- to support the healthy and safe development of children and youth

- To realise their talents and potential by becoming contributing members of their community and society

- Try to know the cause behind the crisis, and you're trying to help. Address acceptable risk and preventive factors for the substance use in each population.

3.1 Principles of Prevention

The prevention principles are:

Defining a Population – A population can be defined by age, gender, race, geography, and institution.

Assessing levels of risks, protection, substance misuse for that population – Risk factors raise the risk of substance misuse, and protectors inhibit the risk of substance misuse in the presence of risk. Danger and protective factors may be divided into domains and defined as important to people, families, friends, colleges, workplaces, and the environment.

Focusing on all risk levels, with special attention to those exposed to high and low Protection – The preventive programs and policies should concentrate on all forms of risk, but specific attention should be paid to a given community. Population evaluation may help to sharpen the preventive emphasis.

Reducing the availability of substances like illicit drugs, alcohol, and tobacco for the under aged – Community regulation, policies and services will limit the supply and marketing of illegal substances. They will also minimize the supply and attractiveness of alcohol and nicotine to the underaged

Strengthening anti-substance use behaviours and norms – Strengthen environmental support for anti-substance use attitudes by exchanging reliable statistics on substances abuse, promoting substance free behaviours and upholding legislation and regulations related to controlled substances.

Strengthening life skills and the methods of substance rejection- Teach life skills and substance refusal skills using immersive strategies that rely on critical thought, communication and social competence.

Reducing vulnerability and improve family security- Families reinforce these skills by setting boundaries, clarifying goals, tracking actions, engaging consistently, offering social reinforcement, and modelling healthy behaviours.

Strengthening the bonding of culture – Strengthen social connections and nurturing relationships for opioid addiction in communities, moral environments, and organised leisure events.

Ensuring that the initiatives are sufficient for the communities to be discussed – Ensure the preventative interventions, including services and policies are suitable and sufficient for communities and societies needs and motivations to be discussed.

Intervention: try to understand when and where substance misuse begins and intervene early. Some suggestions are as follow-

Intervene early at the point of growth and life changes that foresee potential substance misuse- These developmental stages and life changes may include biological, psychological, or social conditions that may raise the risk of substance misuse. If the processes or changes are anticipated or unpredictable, preventive interventions should be handled as quickly as possible.

Strengthening intervention over time-Repeated exposure to clinically accurate and age- appropriate anti-substance use messaging and other strategies will guarantee that the knowledge, values, aspirations, and attitudes learned earlier are maintained over time.

Managing Prevention Programmes are as follow:

Ensuring continuity and coverage of legislation and services- Implementation of preventive strategies, initiatives and messaging for various areas of the population should be coherent, consistent and relevant.

Preparing the employees and volunteers – To ensure that prevention programmes and messages are implemented daily as planned, instruction cean b given on a routine basis to staff and volunteers.

Tracking and assessing the Programmes – To ensure that goals and objectives are accomplished, the initiative's analysis and assessment should be part of the programme's routine execution. When objectives are not met, changes should be made to maximise production.

Effective substance prevention programmes draw on the efforts and resources of our society's multiple sectors, such as the public, students, parents, peers, religious leaders, law enforcement, the medical community, and community leaders. Performance in preventive strategies improvise as diverse segments come together to deliver consistent anti-substance messaging to specific audiences.

3.2 Ideas for Substance Awareness Projects

Discussions: Keep sessions that allow people to learn about, appreciate, and make positive responses to the topics that impact their lives. The topic ideas include drink-drinking or drug driving, underage use, the effect of substance use on individuals and the community and many more.

Fairs and Displays: Keep the prevention of substance trafficking fair in a car park or corridor or anywhere publicity is caught. Creation of educational shows for malls, classrooms, hospitals, businesses, and neighbourhood centres to attract more individuals or programmes in substance awareness initiatives.

Pamphlets: Design and deliver pamphlets on numerous issues relating to the prevention of drug misuse. If inhalant misuse or marijuana is concern in your culture, study the topic, and make it the focus of your paper. You can find assistance in printing your pamphlets from a store, a local printer, or other neighbourhood organisations.

Videos: Try to write a script, record videos, and edit after making a video as part of an education programme. This can be really helpful to raise awareness against the abusive use of drugs and alcohol.

Performances: Write and produce comedy sketches and shows for other pupils, younger ones, neighbourhoods or groups struggling with any aspect of substance addiction.

Conferences: You might plan a conference on drug-free youth and give presentations on different substances and how to say no and live a substance -free life as well as teaching leadership skills.

Media Campaign: You will be able to make public service announcements (PSA) for radio or television and to persuade the local stations to show them. You should submit letters to the editor of your own newspaper. Not only that but you might write an essay on substance addiction for your school newspaper.

Contests: You can organise contest for raising awareness, such as writing or singing. You can also organise arts contests.

Tutoring and Mentoring: Develop a teaching service to help inform your friends or young teenagers about substance misuse.

3.3 Financial Resources

The launch of a community-based opioid prevention programme would not require large sum of money. The important thing to remember is that there are groups eager to assist young people in making a difference in the fight against narcotics. Programmes or civic clubs, neighbourhood watch groups, municipal companies, and other sources of money are all possibilities. Groups can also make money by hosting events such as concerts or exhibiting awareness films.

Chapter 4

Substance Misuse at Workplace

4.0 Introduction

This chapter will discuss the impacts and signs of substance misuse at work and other aspects of it. It is essential to have a substance misuse free workplace for everyone's safety and wellbeing. Topics to be covered are as follow: -

- Substance Misuse at Work
- Impact of Substance Misuse at Work
- Signs of Substance Use at Work
- Employers Role
- Drug Testing at Workplace
- Workplace Culture
- Workplace Awareness

4.1 Substance Misuse at Work

Some patients have illnesses that need prescription medications to help them live a regular life and can't function without them. It is not illegal to take prescription medications at work. However, it is a criminal offence under the Abuse of Drugs Act 1971 that any person intentionally permits the manufacture, delivery, possession, and usage of prohibited drugs in their premises.

Employers also have a general responsibility to protect workers' health and welfare under the health and safety at work Act 1974 (HASAWA) and carry out risk analysis under the Health and Safety at Work Regulations 1999

Workplaces also represent what happens in society. As substance misuse is a major social problem, it is also an issue in the workplace. Both alcohol and illegal drug consumption are diminishing in the United Kingdom, but in recent years there has been an uptick in the use of new psychoactive substances that were formally 'legally strong', including synthetic cannabinoids, which the press calls 'spice'.

The 2017/18 Crime Report for England and Wales found that 4.3 percent of people aged 16 and 59 years of age had recently taken prescription drugs. This percentage has been dropping since a decade ago because a variety of additional substances (legal highs) have been declared illegal in 2016.

Cannabis, followed by cocaine is the most common synthetic drug used. The use of prescription medications is much more prevalent to people who are at work. Approximately 1.5 million people in the United Kingdom are addicted to prescription and over the counter medications. Many of these medications can have a major impact on efficiency, attention, or alertness.

Many people use alcohol or substances to help deal with work related pressures, and if there is a problem with alcohol or substance addition in the workplace, this could be part of broader stress issue. Some types of medications are also used to combat fatigue. And caffeine, a legal and very common substance, may be used to cover the exhaustion induced by overtime at work.

4.2 Impact of Substance Misuse at Work

In the past, inadequate controls of misuse have led to a decline in health and families, increased injury rates, absenteeism, and decreased productivity of people and their teams. It is also beneficial to us to take a proactive approach to the use of medications in the workplace. When a business doesn't manage substance misuse effectively, they then experience.

- A damage reputation

- A lack of productivity

- Accidents which are ranging from minor to fatal

- A loss of morale in the organisation or within a team

- A breakdown in working relationships.

- Potential legal costs

A poorly handled problem will lead to financial difficulties for the person, deterioration of family relationship, and has historically led to unemployment, domestic violence, and homelessness in some situations.

4.3 Signs of Substance Use at Work

When you have questions about an employee dealing with substance misuse, certain signs indicate that an employee is consuming the substance. The following is non exhaustive but thorough list of warning signs of substance misuse at work.

- An inability to carry out work-related duties.

- Inconsistent job performance

- Frequent small accidents

- Lateness

- Numerous unexplained absences (on average, addicts miss ten working days for every one missed by other employees)
- Paranoia and aggression
- Bloodshot eyes or signs of tiredness
- Overreactions to criticism
- Dental problems
- Sudden weight loss/gain
- Unsteady gait
- Bouts of manic activity
- Sluggishness
- Neglecting responsibilities
- Participating in dangerous or criminal behaviours such as disorderly behaviour, carelessness, drink-driving, or theft
- Neglecting or damaging working relationships

4.4 Employer's Role

Employers should take easy measures to defend themselves and their employees such as:

- Recognising the impact of substance misuse on the bottom line

- Educating and engaging their workforce on the topic of opioids

- Enacting clear and strong company substance free workplace policies and ensuring consistence and comprehensive communication with employees

- Expanding drug panel testing to include opioids.

- Training supervisors and employees to spot the first sign signs of substance misuse and impairment.

- Treating substance use disorders as a medical condition that can and should be treated and ensuring evidence-based treatment mechanism are covered by employer health care plans (if applicable)

- Leveraging employee assistant programmes and other similar resources to help employees return to work and supporting employees in recovery.

4.5 Drug Testing at Workplace

Drug monitoring is not recommended but is always a safe practice. This is because it produces scepticism, and a substance user can find ways to trick the process. However, if your field is a high-risk place for substance misuse, you might consider incorporating drug and alcohol monitoring into your substance policies. If you want to make a substance screening part of your policy, you can order a drug and alcohol test kit online. These kits may include.

- A digital breathalyser
- Single-use breath alcohol strip detectors
- Mouthpieces (to use with breathalyser)
- Drug test cups (to screen urine and saliva)

Urine and saliva tests could detect the use of marijuana, cocaine, morphine, amphetamines, benzodiazepines, tramadol, ketamine, methadone, methamphetamine and MDMA. In addition to technology, managers may use visual assessment measures to detect levels of intoxication and impairment.

The field impairment test is often used by police, which includes five assessment measure:

- The pupil measure test looks at the size, condition, and reaction to light of pupils.
- The 'Romberg test' involves standing still, tilting the head backward and counting to 30 seconds to test balance and time judgement.

- The 'work and turn test' may indicate impairment if someone stumbles or steps off the line.
- The 'one leg stand test' evaluates balance.
- The 'finger to nose test' assesses coordination.

4.6 Workplace Culture

The workplace culture can play a major role in whether drinking and using substances are accepted and encouraged or discouraged and inhibited. Part of this culture may depend on the gender mix of employees.

Research in predominantly female occupations shows that male and female employees are less likely to have substance misuse problems that male dominated employees. Studies have shown that male dominated occupations create heavy drinking cultures in which employees drink to build solidarity and show conformity. These occupations, therefore, have higher rates of alcohol related and substance related problems.

6.7 Workplace Awareness

One powerful way to affect workers emotional, physical, economic, and social wellbeing is to foster a health ethic through advertising programmes. Researchers have found that prevention programmes that aim to warn people away from substance use are unsuccessful. Instead, campaigns are more successful in fostering a larger stance on safe living. Your initiative should be basic in the staff room or anywhere the workers want.

A display board with support details can be an easy way to remind staff that there's support. It will also go a long way towards building an atmosphere where staff and service consumers are free to come out and communicate to management about problems.

Chapter 5

Substance Misuse Policy at Workplace

5.0 Introduction

Having a well-defined policy about substance misuse can help the people engaged in the workplace stay safe. In this chapter we will talk about creating a policy at the workplace to prevent substance misuse. Topics to be covered are as follow:

- Understanding Policies to mitigate Harms in the United Kingdom
- Substance Misuse Policy
- Aims and Objectives
- Developing a Policy on Substances at Workplace
- Negotiation of Policy
- Major Elements of Policy

5.1 Understanding Policies to Mitigate Harms in the United Kingdom

A significant body of research suggests that tailored and population-wide alcohol restriction measures can mitigate alcohol-related damage. Historically, shifts in alcohol regulation laws in the United Kingdom have been followed by variations in the level of alcohol intake and related issues.

In the 18th Century, a drastic rise in gin use occurred in the United Kingdom after a decrease in tax prices, leading to an era of

- Severe chronic alcoholism
- Drunken abuse
- Illness
- Alcohol dependency
- Premature mortality

During the first and second world wars and the inter-war period, some measures were taken which helped with the issues related to alcohol consumption. Those measures are-

- Bans on the selling of alcohol drinks.
- Increased taxes

Reducing the impact of substance misuse in the United Kingdom requires good leadership and the adoption of successful alcohol regulation measures that limit total intake levels and mitigate risks to the public and individuals. The implementation of effective substance management programmes also involves a collaboration between government departments and organisations throughout the United Kingdom. A coordinated strategy is also needed to increase the public's visibility and approval of such policies.

5.2 Substance Misuse Police

A company has its own policy. Many of these policies are identical. If you review policies against substance used in the workplace, you can find some typical challenges described in the policies. Those are as follow-

- Purpose
- Scope
- Policy
- Definition of Substance Misuse
- Principles
- Identification of Substance Misuse
- Substances at Work
- Policy Review
- Relevant Legislation

The new drug policy lays out how the government can handle the complicated problem of drug addiction. Strides have been made in recent years, but problems persist, including rising rates of substance-related deaths

5.3 Aims and Objectives

The policy should be seen in the context of a desire to promote all employees' general well-being. It should be designed to:

- Provide a structure for the effective and consistent treatment of drugs, alcohol, and substance misuse cases. It should lay down guidelines on the use of intoxicating drugs to ensure that workers are mindful.

- Prevent accidents and impaired performance at work that may be related to alcohol or drugs, ensuring the safety and well-being of staff and patients.

- To actively enhance knowledge and understanding of the impact of substance misuse related issues on the workplace. Also, to highlight the possible consequences of such misuse on peoples' health and work and enable those with challenges to seek support.

5.4 Developing a Policy on Substances at Workplace

Employers are responsible for ensuring the health and welfare of their workers. A decent boss would still try to support those workers who have a drug or alcohol addiction. That is why it is critical for any employer to have a policy on drugs and alcohol. Two different issues nee to be considered in every policy on drugs and alcohol.

The first is the issue of drugs at work. Anyone under the influence of any drug or alcohol that may affect their ability is likely to be at risk to themselves and others. This is especially the case in high hazard sectors and extends almost as well to some prescription drugs as to illicit substances.

The second is the effect of a person's dependence on alcohol. This may have an impact on their results but may also have a long-term impact on their health and finances. Some employers view drug use outside the workplace as a matter of law, and substance misuse is also considered a personal matter until it appears to be harmful. Negotiating a negotiated policy will help ensure that problems are dealt with as valid job issues in a manner that is intended to benefit any worker who has a concern. Drugs or alcohol policy can in no condition be part of a discipline policy.

Management and employees must be both mindful of how the company can cope with drug and alcohol-related problems. Unfortunately, many line managers are not trained to deal with these problems, and preparation and support for line managers is an important aspect of any policy. It is recommended to employers that when they become aware of issues like drug and alcohol misuse, they should:

- Keep accurate, confidential records of instances of poor performance or other problems.
- Interview the worker in private as early as possible in the process.
- Concentrate on the instances of poor performance that have been identified.
- Ask for the employee's reasons for poor performance and question whether it could be due to a health problem, without explicitly mentioning alcohol or drugs.

- If appropriate, discuss your alcohol and drugs policy and the help available inside or outside your organisation.
- Agree with future action.
- Arrange regular meetings to monitor progress and discuss any further problems if they arise.

However, this must be achieved within the context of an established policy on drugs and alcohol, which all employees are informed of. Where certain laws fail, there is a need to offer concrete support to those who have a problem. Employers would need to provide some sort of plan to assist staff classified as in need of assistance.

5.5 Negotiation of Policy

It is best to figure out what issues exists before developing a strategy. This can be done by looking at the illness and administrative history, the injury investigation files, or referring to the workplace health professional where they exist. However, even though there is no evidence of a concern, you should advise your company to create a strategy. The policy should set out it aims, including:

- The recognition that substance misuse is both a health problem and a safety problem.

- That substance misuse should be prevented by increasing awareness of the issue and changing the organisation's culture.

- That those employees with a problem should be identified at an early stage

- That assistance should be offered to those with a substance related problem.

5.6 Major Elements of Policy

Any policy should address the following issues:

- It should make it clear who has ultimate responsibility for the implementation of the policy.

- This would protect all legal and illegal drugs.

- Both staff, including senior management, should be protected by the regulation.

- The employer should ensure that all employees requesting assistance are handled in a non-judgemental and compassionate manner, and that secrecy is assured.

- It should lay down processes for the dealing with any cases when someone is believed to be impaired by drug or alcohol while at work and outline when, it at all, alcohol can be consumed while at work or on work premises.

- It should ensure that all employees are qualified to identify early signs of harassment and processes that in place to ensure that any issues are addressed with workers at an early level.

- Alcohol and substance addiction should be viewed as a medical and not criminal matter. Besides, it can also be remembered that in any situations, alcohol and substance consumption can lead to addiction and will need assistance.

- If drug or alcohol testing is to be used as part of a drugs and alcohol policy, it should be restricted to safety reasons, and employees should be aware of their rights.

- The policy should explain how employees will obtain help within the organisation and, and if necessary, outside the organisation.

- It should be emphasised that all demands for help of care would be handled confidentially.

- The supervisor should consider finding substitute jobs possible, where this allows the employee to be rehabilitated.
- The policy should make it clear that absence for treatment and rehabilitation will be regarded as normal sickness absence.
- It should be understood that workers can relapse.
- The policy should outline the conditions in which corrective action can be taken and this can include where support is denied; besides, performance is regularly low due to drug or alcohol addictions, or where an employee comes to work under the influence of drugs or alcohol, and others are at risk.
- The employer should undertake to run an information and awareness campaign in support of the policy.

It is also important that any policy is regularly monitored and reviewed.

Chapter 6

Treatment of Substance Addition

6.0 Prevention and Awareness

Introduction: Substance misuse can have far reaching implications. In this chapter you will learn about the prevention principles and methods that could be relevant solutions. Topics to be covered are as follow:

Why is Prevention Important?

Principles of Prevention

- Intervention
- Managing Prevention Programs

Ideas for Substance Awareness Projects

- Discussions
- Fairs and Displays
- Pamphlets
- Videos
- Performances
- Media Campaign
- Conferences
- Other Projects

Financial Resources

6.1 Why Is Prevention Important?

Substance abuse is a leading source of sickness and mortality in the world. In addition, substance abuse can have severe repercussions and worsen existing individual and social inequities.

Substance abuse can lead to a decline in physical and mental health and social issues on an individual level. Therefore, a comprehensive approach to manage substance use and support the population's health, well-being and productivity must include prevention. It is especially crucial in rural areas, where many young people and adolescents are marginalised and poor. Evidence based preventative methods that are implemented over time and address various age groups and communities can have a significant impact on rural youths and adolescents' health and well-being.

The primary goal of substance use prevention is to help non substance users avoid or delay substance use initiation. For those who are already substance users, prevention seeks to minimise the likelihood of developing substance use disorders (example, dependence). The prevention also has a broader purpose:

- to support the healthy and safe development of children and youth
- To realise their talents and potential by becoming contributing members of their community and society
- Try to know the cause behind the crisis, and you're trying to help. Address acceptable risk and preventive factors for the substance use in a given population.

6.2 Principles of Prevention

The prevention principles are:

Defining a Population – A population can be defined by age, gender, race, geography, and institution.

Assessing levels of risks, protection, substance misuse for that population – Risk factors raise the risk of substance misuse, and protectors inhibit the risk of substance misuse in the presence of risk. Danger and protective factors may be divided into domains and defined as important to people, families, friends, colleges, workplaces, and the environment.

Focusing on all risk levels, with special attention to those exposed to high and low Protection – The preventive programs and policies should concentrate on all forms of risk, but specific attention should be paid to a given community. Population evaluation may help to sharpen the preventive emphasis.

Reducing the availability of substances like illicit drugs, alcohol, and tobacco for the under aged – Community regulation, policies and services will limit the supply and marketing of illegal substances. They will also minimize the supply and attractiveness of alcohol and nicotine to the underaged

Strengthening anti-substance use behaviours and norms – Strengthen environmental support for anti-substance use attitudes by exchanging reliable statistics on substances abuse, promoting substance free behaviours and upholding legislation and regulations related to controlled substances.

Strengthening life skills and the methods of substance rejection- Teach life skills and substance refusal skills using immersive strategies that rely on critical thought, communication and social competence.

Reducing vulnerability and improve family security- Families reinforce these skills by setting boundaries, clarifying goals, tracking actions, engaging consistently, offering social reinforcement, and modelling healthy behaviours.

Strengthening the bonding of culture – Strengthen social connections and nurturing relationships for opioid addiction in communities, moral environments and organised leisure events.

Ensuring that the initiatives are sufficient for the communities to be discussed – Ensure the preventative interventions, including services and policies are suitable and sufficient for communities and societies needs and motivations to be discussed.

Intervention: try to understand when and where substance misuse begins and intervene early. Some suggestions are as follow-

Intervene early at the point of growth and life changes that foresee potential substance misuse- These developmental stages and life changes may include biological, psychological, or social conditions that may raise the risk of substance misuse. If the processes or changes are anticipated or unpredictable, preventive interventions should be handled as quickly as possible.

Strengthening intervention over time-Repeated exposure to clinically accurate and age- appropriate anti-substance use messaging and other strategies will guarantee that the knowledge, values, aspirations, and attitudes learned earlier are maintained over time.

Managing Prevention Programmes are as follow:

Ensuring continuity and coverage of legislation and services- Implementation of preventive strategies, initiatives, and messaging for various areas of the population should be coherent, consistent and relevant.

Preparing the employees and volunteers – To ensure that prevention programmes and messages are implemented on a daily basis as planned, instruction ca b given on a routine basis to staff and volunteers.

Tracking and assessing the Programmes – To ensure that goals and objectives are accomplished, the initiative's analysis and assessment should be part of the programme's routine execution. When objectives are not met, changes should be made to maximise production.

Effective substance prevention programmes draw on the efforts and resources of our society's multiple sectors, such as the public, students, parents, peers, religious leaders, law enforcement, the medical community, and community leaders. Performance in preventive strategies improvise as diverse segments come together to deliver consistent anti-substance messaging to specific audiences.

6.3 Ideas for Substance Awareness Projects

Discussions: Keep sessions that allow people to learn about, appreciate, and make positive responses to the topics that impact their lives. The topic ideas include drink-drinking or drug driving, underage use, the effect of substance use on individuals and the community and many more.

Fairs and Displays: Keep the prevention of substance trafficking fair in a car park or corridor or anywhere publicity is caught. Creation of educational shows for malls, classrooms, hospitals, businesses, and neighbourhood centres to attract more individuals or programmes in substance awareness initiatives.

Pamphlets: Design and deliver pamphlets on numerous issues relating to the prevention of drug misuse. If inhalant misuse or marijuana is concern in your culture, study the topic, and make it the focus of your paper. You can find assistance in printing your pamphlets from a store, a local printer, or other neighbourhood organisations.

Videos: Try to write a script, record videos, and edit after making a video as part of an education programme. This can be really helpful to raise awareness against the abusive use of drugs and alcohol.

Performances: Write and produce comedy sketches and shows for other pupils, younger ones, neighbourhoods or groups struggling with any aspect of substance addiction.

Conferences: You might plan a conference on drug-free youth and give presentations on different substances and how to say no and live a substance -free life as well as teaching leadership skills.

Media Campaign: You will be able to make public service announcements (PSA) for radio or television and to persuade the local stations to show them. You should submit letters to the editor of your own newspaper. Not only that but you might write an essay on substance addiction for your school newspaper.

Contests: You can organise contest for raising awareness, such as writing or singing. You can also organise arts contests.

Tutoring and Mentoring: Develop a teaching service to help inform your friends or young teenagers about substance misuse.

6.4 Financial Resources

The launch of a community-based opioid prevention programme would not require large sum of money. The important thing to remember is that there are groups eager to assist young people in making a difference in the fight against narcotics. Programmes or civic clubs, neighbourhood watch groups, municipal companies, and other sources of money are all possibilities. Groups can also make money by hosting events such as concerts or exhibiting awareness films.

Chapter 7

Laws and Act on Substances

Laws and legislation can play a huge role in deducting the amount of substance misuse and prevent the spread of it. In this chapter focuses on the laws and legislations regarding drugs and substance misuse. Topics to be covered as follow:

- Introduction
- The Misuse of Drugs Act (2001)
- Penalties
- Regulations
- The Medicines Act (1968)
- The Psychoactive Substance Act (2016)
- Other Relevant Laws

7.0 Introduction

It is not just the drug dealers who are going to be arrested if they get caught. Carrying drugs for personal use might give you a big fine or time in jail too. So it's a safe thing to consider the rules on the classification, distribution and purpose of drugs. The laws controlling drug use are complicated. The penalties depend on the type of drug or substance, the amount you have in your possession and whether you're also dealing or producing. There are three main statutes regulating the availability of drugs in the United Kingdom:

- The Misuse of Drugs Act (2001)
- The Medicines Act (1968)
- The Psychoactive Substance Act (2016)

7.1 The Misuse of Drugs Act (2001)

Although much of this Act consolidated older laws, it made several significant reforms. The purpose of this act is to prohibit the non-medicinal usage of medication. For this purpose, it regulates medicinal medications (which would now be part of the Medicines Act) and drugs of no current medical usage. Drugs that are subject to this act are classified as controlled drugs.

The statute specifies the number of offences, including unlawful procurement, intention to supply, import or export and unlawful production. The Misuse of Drugs Regulations 2001, created under the Act 2001 Act are about licences classified under the Act. The biggest distinction from the Medicines Act is that the Misuse of Drugs Act still forbids illegal possession of drugs. In order to enforce this law, the police have to stop, arrest and search people on 'reasonable suspicion' that they are in possession of controlled drugs. The Misuse of Drugs Act (MDA) separates drugs into three classes. They are as follow:

Class A: This includes: -

- Cocaine and Crack
- Ecstasy
- MDMA (added in January 2021)
- Heroin
- LSD
- Methadone
- Methamphetamine (crystal meth)
- Freshly prepared magic mushrooms

Class B: Drugs in this class are: -

- Amphetamine
- Barbiturates
- Codeine
- Ketamine
- Mephedrone
- Methylone

- MDPV

- Synthetic Cannabinoids such as spice and cannabis (medicinal cannabis can be prescribed by doctors from 1 November 2018)

Class C: These include: -

- Anabolic Steroids

- Khat

- Piperazines (BZP)

- Gamma-butyrolactone (GBL)

- Gamma hydroxybutyrate (GHB)

- Minor tranquilisers or benzodiazepines

The government can ban new drugs for a year under 'temporary prohibition order' while deciding how to classify the drugs. Class A Drugs are treated as the most dangerous by statute. Crimes under the Misuse of Drugs Act can include:

- Possession of illegal drugs

- Possession with the intention of providing another user.

- Production, cultivation, or production of controlled substances

- Supplying someone else with controlled substances

- Offering the supply of managed drugs to another user

- Importing or exporting controlled substances

- Allowing premises that you occupy or manage to use for the use of such regulated substances (smoking cannabis or heroin while not using other controlled drugs) or for the purchase or manufacture of other controlled drugs.

- Certain controlled substances, such as amphetamines, barbiturates, methadone, mild tranquilisers and even heroin, can be obtained through a legal doctor's prescription. In such circumstances, their holdings is not unlawful

Temporary Class Drug Orders

On 15 November 2011, the Misuse Of Drugs Act 1971 was amended to enable the Home Secretary to put a new psychoactive drug, which isn't controlled as Class A, B, or C drug but causes alarm, under provisional supervision by invoking a temporary class drug orders. The Temporary Class Drugs Order (TCDO) comes into effect immediately and lasts for up to twelve months. This duration gives the advisory council on Drug Misuse (ACDM) time to offer professional guidance on the temporary class of drugs and their associated harms.

The TCDO shall be subject to parliamentary scrutiny at or at the conclusion of the twelve-month term. After twelve months, the TCDO will expire unless it is permanently regulated by the Misuse of Drugs Act 1971 or extended. Offences committed under the 2001 Act in relation to a temporary class drug are subject to the following maximum penalties:

- 14 years imprisonment and an unlimited fine or indictment
- 6 months imprisonment and a £5,000 fine on summary

Simple possession of temporary class drug is not an offence under the 2001 Act.

Alcohol

Providing alcohol to a child under five years of age, either in an emergency or under medical care (children and young persons Act 1933) is an offence. It is also an offence for a vendor to knowingly sell alcohol to an individual under the age of 18 and to purchase alcohol under the age of 18. A 16-year-old will drink beer or wine in a pub while enjoying a meal in an area set aside for this reason with the supervision of an individual over 18 years old

Tobacco and Tranquillisers

It is a crime for a vendor to market tobacco goods to someone they suspect is under the age of 18. Tobacco products must be sold in their original packaging, and it is illegal to sell single cigarettes to any person, adult, or child. Smoking in public places has been prohibited in the United Kingdom since 1 July 2007. Minor tranquillisers are controlled as class C drugs under the Misuse of Drugs Act. The maximum penalty is two years or fine or both for possession of it. It is an offence to sell or deliver them to another human.

Poppers

Liquid gold, amyl or butyl nitrites are known as poppers. They are not covered by the MDA and are not illegal to possess or buy. They are mostly available in joke and sex shops but often some bars, clubs, tobacconists, and occasionally music or clothing stores used by young people.

Although not thoroughly checked in court, the Medicines Control Agency has confirmed that poppers are considered to be medicinal products and thus come under some scope of the Medicines Act 1968

Solvents

Solvents are aerosols, gases, glues and many more. They are not illegal to possess, use or buy at any age. In England and Wales, it is an offence for shopkeeper to distribute them to people under 18 years of age if they know they are to be used for intoxicating purposes. The government has expanded this law to make it illegal for shopkeepers to sell lighter fuel (butane) to those under the age of 18, whether they realise it would be used for intoxicating purposes.

Anabolic Steroids

These drugs are controlled under the Misuse of Drugs Act as class C drugs, but their legal status is complicated. In most cases, possession offences are waived, ensuring that those who carry or use steroids without a prescription are unlikely to be charged. However, in some parts of the United Kingdom, police have effectively arrested individuals for possession of steroids are not in the content of a pharmaceutical substance. It is often an offence to sell or supply steroids to another person. People can also be arrested for possession with the intention to distribute if they have significant amounts of steroids without a prescription for them.

7.2 Penalties

Maximum Penalties under the Misuse of Drugs Act are given below:

Drug Class	Possession	Supply
++--Class A	7 Years + Fine	Life + Fine
Class B	5 Years + Fine	14 Years + Fine
Class C	2 Years + Fine	14 Years + Fine

Maximum penalties vary depending on the type of offence. Fewer for possession, more for dealing in manufacturing or allowing a property to be used for the manufacture or supply of narcotics. They also differ depending on how dangerous the drug is considered to be. Less violent crimes are normally dealt with by magistrates court, where fines cannot reach six months or a fine of £5,00 or three months. Any opioid user is guilty of illegal possession. While the maximum sentences are serious, only about one in five persons guilty of possession receives a custody term, and even fewer ultimately go to jail, with a number of fines of £50 or less.

Regulations

Most controlled substances have medical applications, some may be of research significance, so the Act requires the government to allow the purchase, supply, manufacture and import or export of substances to meet medical or science needs. These exemptions to the general prohibitions are rendered in the form of regulations under the Act.

The most limited drugs can only be distributed or possessed for testing or other special uses by people authorised by the Home Office. These substances are not eligible for regular medicinal use and cannot be used by physicians who do not have a licence. All other medications are available for routine medical use.

7.3 The Medicines Act (1968)

This law governs the manufacture and supply of medicine.
It divides medical drugs into three categories which are:

- Prescription Only Medicines: These are the most restricted. They can only be sold or supplied by a pharmacist if supplied by a doctor.
- Pharmacy Medicines: These can be sold without a prescription but only by a pharmacist
- General Sales List Medicines: The medicines under this category can be sold by any shop, not just a pharmacy.

The enforcement of the Medicines Act rarely affects the public. On 14 August 2012, Section 10(7) of the Medicines Act 1968 was repealed. Section 10(7) provided an exemption in the United Kingdom law from a pharmacist's requirement to hold a wholesale Dealer's Licence if they trade in medicines in certain circumstances.

7.4 The Psychoactive Substances Act (2016)

The psychoactive substances Act received Royal Assent on 28 January 2016. The Act applied across the United Kingdom and came into force on 26 May 2016. The Act:

- Makes it an offence to produce, supply, offer to supply, possess with intent to supply, posses on custodial premises, import or export psychoactive substances; that is, any substance intended for human consumption that is capable of producing a psychoactive effect. The maximum sentence will be seven years imprisonment.

- Excludes legitimate substances, such as food, alcohol, tobacco, nicotine, caffeine, and medical products from the scope of the offence, as well as controlled drugs, which continue to be regulated by the Misuse of Drugs Act 1971

- Exempts healthcare activities and approved scientific research from the offences under the Act on the basis that persons engaged in such activities have a legitimate need to use psychoactive substances in their work

- Includes provision for civil sanction – prohibition notices, premises notices, prohibition orders and premises orders (breach of the two orders will be a criminal offence) – to enable the police and local authorities to adopt a graded response to the supply of psychoactive substances in appropriate cases

- Provides powers to stop and search persons, vehicles and vessels, enter and search premises in accordance with warrant, and to seize and destroy psychoactive substances.

Other Relevant Laws:

7.5 Customs and Excise Management Act, 1979

The customs and Excise Act punishes the unauthorised manufacture or sale of regulated drugs. Maximum sentences shall be the same as for all narcotics crimes, provided that fines can be up to three times the amount of substances confiscated by a court of magistrates. The importation or exportation of any controlled drug is prohibited unless it is done in accordance with the terms of a licence.

7.6 Crime and Disorder Act, 1998

For the first time, this Act introduces enforcement drug treatment and testing orders for people convicted of crimes committed to maintaining their drug use.

7.7 Road Traffic Act, 1972

It is an offence to b in possession of a motor vehicle whilst unfit to drive under the influence of a drink or drug. Drugs may include illicit drugs, prescription medicines or solvents. A new offence was introduced in March 2015, which sets the blood concentration thresholds on such substances. This does not substitute all previous driving

offences with drugs that are affected like legal
medications.

Drug Traffic Act, 1994

It is an offence to supply articles to prepare or administer
controlled substances such as cocaine snorting kits. The
Act also provides for the prosecution of properties and
profits of a person found guilty of drug trafficking, even
though the assets and income cannot be proven to have
been derived from the proceeds of drug trafficking.